LIVING ⟨barcode: D1650735⟩

Written by an angina ⟨…⟩ this book explains how to cope with the illness and live as full a life as possible. It describes the workings of the heart and how angina is caused, and the method of treatment by diet and relaxation which has helped the author. Finally, it shows how the angina patient can adapt his working and home conditions for maximum activity and independence, and how his family can best deal with the situation.

LIVING WITH ANGINA

by

R. WILLIAM THOMSON

NATURE'S WAY

THORSONS PUBLISHERS LIMITED
Wellingborough, Northamptonshire

First published June 1976
Second Impression December 1976
Third Impression 1979
Fourth Impression 1981

ISBN 0 7225 0338 5 (paperback)
ISBN 0 7225 0364 4 (hardback)

Photoset by
Specialised Offset Services Ltd., Liverpool.
Printed and bound in Great Britain
by Richard Clay (The Chaucer Press), Ltd.,
Bungay, Suffolk.

CONTENTS

CHAPTER ONE

'SO, I HAVE ANGINA'

I suppose that I largely brought it on myself. I had for many years pushed myself and others too hard. I was the type who was never really satisfied with what had been done, a worrier with an ambition to succeed. To get to work I travelled, crushed like a sardine, in a crowded tube train. Every screech of the wheels threw a further stress on mind and body. At work I became very irritated if a secretary mislaid a letter, or a phone call interrupted an important conversation. In the evenings I sat down at home with a bulging brief case and continued to work. At weekends I wrote educational text books. Even on holiday, unless I was abroad, work would be sent on to me – letters which needed advice if they were to be properly answered, proofs for correction. When I was about fifty, I began to put on weight, amounting to three stone in a few years. A wise and loving wife continually begged me to ease up and leave more to others. Most of the time, I ignored that advice.

Then came the first flashes of a red light – a kind of discomfort in the chest which did not appear to be due to indigestion. It could be described as a feeling of tightness across the chest, but not created by a cold or cough. And then an ache in the left arm, a nagging, irritating ache. Also a shortness of breath which began to grow more acute when, say, gardening. My son, home from abroad and helping me in the garden one day, turned to me and asked, 'Father, are you developing asthma?'

Eventually, I went to see my local G.P., and was sent to a Harley Street heart specialist. The diagnosis was, as it were, broken to me in stages. I had hardening of the arteries. I had a cardiac insufficiency. What did that mean? Not enough blood was reaching the heart at some stages in my day and my activities. Finally, I was told I had angina, but not severely. There seemed to be an unspoken feeling that the word 'angina' had better be kept from me as it was an emotive word with horrific connotations. I came away from the consulting room, not appalled, but saying, 'So, I have angina'. I hoped to live with it quite comfortably.

And so I could have done, I expect. But unfortunate circumstances closed in on me. Changes in staff, shortage of staff, problems that caused some colleagues to come and cry on my shoulder, proved very worrying. More and more work. The result was that the pain came more often and more severely after a time, and finally I could go on no longer. I was obliged to retire some eighteen months before the normal age. I was faced with a new sort of life, a good deal of pain on the slightest extra effort, and many worries.

THE SYMPTOMS OF ANGINA

'Angina pectoris' is the full name of this heart ailment. The name literally means 'pain in the chest', and that describes it very well. The term is used to describe a pain which results from the heart muscle receiving less blood than it needs for the work which it is being asked to do. We all know how a muscle will complain if put under undue stress – our muscles ache after the first game of tennis in the season, when new stresses have been put on them! In angina, the heart warns gently at first that it is under strain, but if the warnings are ignored the pain may, and usually does, increase in severity. We shall see in a later chapter why this happens. At the moment we are dealing with the symptoms of angina.

At first the discomfort is felt in unusual circumstances – running for a bus, perhaps. There may be nothing to alarm us. A person may hurry up a steep hill and feel more than usually breathless. An ache develops in his chest, he pauses to rest, and the pain goes away.

In time the pain may come on more frequently and with the slightest extra exertion. This may take place months, or even years, after the first signs have been noticed. The description sometimes used for this ailment, 'angina of effort', again describes it very exactly. A commuter hurries to catch his train on a cold morning; he may be overweight, there may be an incline up to the station, or stairs up to the platform. He notices a tightness in his chest and a pain. He tries to hurry on and the pain gets worse until he sinks exhausted into his seat on the train. If he sits quietly the pain dies away after a time, but leaves him feeling limp. If he ignores the pain and hurries on, he may reach a state of collapse.

The typical angina pain is in the front of the chest, and perhaps the shoulders, and it may affect the back of the neck. It usually radiates down the left arm. It may be accompanied by breathlessness. People describe the pain in various ways – as an ache, a constriction across the chest, a tightness, a feeling of oppression. One person said it felt like a ton weight on the chest. And it comes on with effort, lasts for several minutes and will die away if the patient rests quietly.

A SIGNAL TO STOP

The patient has to realize that angina pain is a signal to stop and rest. This is how it differs from that of a coronary thrombosis. The pain of the latter may be fairly similar but more intense, and it can come on whilst at rest, or wake the patient in the night. It does not disappear on relaxing. Angina pain is sometimes thought to be indigestion. An ulcer in the stomach or duodenum, or gastritis, may produce similar symptoms of pain, but it is more of an abdominal discomfort, pain or cramp, and is often associated with vomiting. These are not heart symptoms. Angina pain is usually felt in the chest, arms and neck. As has been said already, it feels like a great pressure on the chest, a tightness, a squeezing, a load.

It helps to realize that one is not unique in having angina – indeed, heart ailments are more common than ever before, for reasons we shall examine later. It is important to realize also that one is not going to be condemned to spend the rest of one's life in a chronic state of invalidism. Our grandparents may have regarded the verdict 'angina pectoris' as a death sentence, and there is some lingering memory of this in us all. Perhaps they were right in their day. But today much help is available, and a great deal of it has to be self-help. And with that help most of us with angina can lead a pretty full and satisfying life, as I have proved.

REASSURANCE

No one would decry the work of family doctors, or hospitals. And yet, kind as they were to me, I felt something lacking. I think this can best be summed up as 'reassurance', or perhaps simply 'information'. Naturally, when one's body gets out of order it becomes a matter of acute personal interest. Most people today, with a wider education giving a knowledge of many scientific and medical matters, are reluctant just to deliver themselves to doctors to be poked about, prodded and consulted over, and treated without any real explanation as to what is going on. People want to know what is wrong, why it is wrong, and how it can be put right or its worst effects avoided.

This outlook is not unreasonable, nor is it a sign of 'invalidism'. Medicine is no longer a mystic art, and the doctor a high-priest. But the kind of relationship we would like to have with a doctor is hard to achieve. Some rare doctors pull it off. But as one family doctor wrote about the National Health Service, in the *Daily Telegraph* on 8 May 1975: 'It is easy to *manage* 3000 patients but it is quite impossible to *doctor* them, to *listen* to them, to examine them, and *reassure* them, as we were taught as students.' (The italics are mine.) The doctor goes on to say that the G.P. needs to give almost ten times as much time to examination and reassurance as he normally allows each patient.

The pressures of today on doctor and on hospital do not allow for this, though one notes from a recent report that St James's Hospital,

Leeds, is issuing patients in the orthopaedic department with tapes which answer the questions so many ask, and give basic information about treatment and so on. This is a step forward, but a tape recording is far removed from a friendly personality answering your own questions.

NATUROPATHIC HELP

Fortunately, there are others who can help. The practising naturopath often has far more time for his patients. I found much to help me in his advice and his treatment. And being one who has spent much of his time reducing complicated facts to fairly simple text books for schools, I have tried to do my part to help fellow sufferers. I read all I could about angina, consulted doctors and naturopaths, and talked to others who are learning how to manage with their ailment. What I now present from these sources will perhaps be worthy of consideration. It is not a text book on cardio-vascular troubles. I am only a layman in all these matters. But illness sharpens the wits sometimes and one seeks to learn about one's ills. And sometimes a layman acting as a kind of 'medical journalist' can interpret the things others have discovered in such a way that everyone is helped. That is my hope. I can report a large measure of success with myself. When I came to premature retirement, my angina was severe. I could not dress or shave without pain, and had to rest to allow it to ease. Four years later I can hold down a small part-time job, do a little gardening, and some easy interior decorating.

Let us be very clear: *Angina is an ailment where*

self-understanding and a careful regime of self-treatment is essential. In few other ailments, except perhaps diabetes, does so much depend upon the patient understanding what triggers off his trouble and why, and how to avoid it.

There are too many half truths and old wives' tales about. Misinformation does not help any of us to adopt the careful and optimistic regime which can help us to enjoy life even though we have angina. This book may help others not to resent the angina pain, but to make friends with the heart and circulation, and make the very best of life.

CHAPTER TWO

HOW THE HEART WORKS

Put your hand on the left side of your chest and you will feel your heart beating. With average health it will beat seventy times a minute for seventy years, so that in the average life span it will beat about two and a half million times. It is the most fantastic pump ever built, although only as big as your fist. It pumps 2000 gallons of blood every twenty-four hours, causing the blood to circulate around a closed line of 'tubes'. Between beats the heart is relaxed and fills with blood. Then the muscular walls contract and eject the contents. The heart beats more quickly when we do a strenuous job, because more blood is needed in order to undertake the new task. In the same way, excitement, fear or anxiety can cause the heart to beat faster. Some illnesses will also do this.

Here is a simple sketch of the heart, and a

simplified explanation of the way it works:

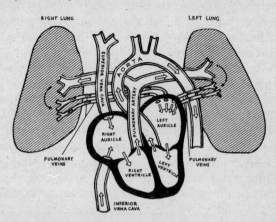

The heart is like two self-contained rooms side by side, and each contains two pumping units. This allows the heart to receive and send out two separate streams of blood.

LIFE-GIVING STREAM

Something should be said here about this life-giving stream. We all know what blood looks like, but are not always clear about its composition and its purpose. It is composed of a sticky fluid called plasma. This is a solution of proteins and minerals in which are floating a number of minute blood cells or corpuscles. These are of two kinds – red (which give the blood its colour) and white. A cubic millimetre of blood contains about five million red and 5000 white corpuscles. Their chief function is to take up oxygen from the air in the lungs and carry it to the tissues. Blood circulates throughout the body and conveys food and oxygen to every part of it, and it also carries away waste products from the tissues and these are discharged from the body through the excretory organs. Too few red blood cells spell anaemia.

After it has done its job in every part of the body, the blood enters the right side of the heart, where it collects in the auricle. It now contains little oxygen.

The four pumping units beat in unison. Valves prevent the blood flowing the wrong way. At the start of each heartbeat the two auricles push open the valves and empty the blood into the ventricles. They give a big push and the blood is thrust out. On the right side it is pushed along into the lungs. It travels along the pulmonary artery which has thick walls designed to stretch and withstand the pressure. The lungs give the blood the oxygen it requires for its work, and stale gasses are released. The blood is refreshed and cleansed – in somewhat the same way that oil in a car is cleaned when it goes through the oil filter.

The blood flows back to the heart, this time to the left side. Again it collects in the auricle, before entering the ventricle and being pumped out to the body. This time the artery is a very big one called the aorta. It feeds the blood to all the organs and tissues of the body. Within two minutes of leaving the heart every ejection of blood (about a wine-glass full) has travelled the whole journey round the circulation system and is back to the heart.

NERVE IMPULSES

The orderly working of the heart is controlled by nerve impulses from a control centre in the brain. These nerve impulses can be measured by the electro-cardiograph. Two or three wires are attached to different parts of the patient's body, and the electrical impulses are picked up and recorded on a moving photographic strip. The patient, by the way, feels no discomfort.

The heart and the whole circulatory system are controlled by the nervous system of the body. When any part of the body feels the need for extra blood, the control system (receiving messages from every organ and every part of the body) assesses the need, as it were, and sends a message to regulate the blood vessels, thus supplying the need. The force of the blood rushing through the arteries and veins is called the blood-pressure and can be accurately measured. It reaches a peak as each new ejection of blood is pumped from the heart, then the pressure gradually fades away to a point where it is at its lowest before the next heartbeat. The first is called the systolic pressure and the second the diastolic.

BLOOD-PRESSURE

Blood-pressure was first measured some 200 years ago by an English clergyman, the Reverend Stephen Hales. He worked out his experiments on a horse! The first practical instrument for use on humans was devised by an Italian doctor, Scipione Riva-Rocci, in 1896. We have probably all had our blood-pressure measured – the rubber cuff is placed around the upper arm and inflated, and a column of mercury rises in the instrument to record the systolic and the diastolic pressure. The doctor uses his stethoscope, which is placed over the main artery at the elbow, in order to note when the sound of blood being stopped by the pressure disappears and reappears. The instrument for measuring blood-pressure is called a sphygmomanometer.

Everyone has blood-pressure. It is incorrect for some people to say that they suffer from blood-pressure when what they mean is that they have a higher blood-pressure than normal.

The blood, as we have seen, is pumped down the aorta, which is gradually turned away into branches leading to limbs and organs. The main branches break up into smaller ones, and so it goes on. One of the few places where an artery lies near the surface is at the wrist, below the root of the thumb. By feeling the pulse here, the number of heartbeats a minute can be counted. And the strength of the pulse tells of the health of the circulation. The average pulse rate is seventy, but a resting person may have a lower rate. The rate is also affected by exercise and by emotional stress.

CHANGING FLOW

The body is constantly changing the amount of blood flow to meet immediate needs. As we have seen, the nerve centre controls this flow Changes are made not only to meet the needs, say, of sudden movement — but also to meet changes of temperature. As we know, the body temperature is around 98.6 degrees Fahrenheit. This temperature is held more or less constant by the body and all the body systems are arranged to work best at this temperature.

When we go into a very cold atmosphere, or into a very hot one, the body has to adjust so as to get the inner temperature as near normal as possible. When we shiver in the cold, this is caused by the rapid contraction of muscles. This produces heat which warms up the body. When we are too hot the body compensates by radiating heat from the surface of the skin. The blood flow to the skin increases, carrying body heat to the surface blood vessels, from which it can be radiated. We perspire and this allows the body to lose heat.

Both the person exposed to cold and the person bathed in unusual warmth are asking the body and therefore the heart to work harder. The heart can normally manage this without trouble. It is a skilled pump and can deal with a good deal of extra work. Its reserve capacity is enormous. When playing tennis, we may need four or five times the flow of blood compared with when we are sitting in a chair. The heart will give us this by increasing the number of beats and the flow. But supposing things are not normal?

One of the crucial links in all this chain of command and response is the circulatory system. It was the famous William Harvey who discovered the circulation of the blood in 1628. Even he did not realize the enormous load the arteries have to take. And unfortunately arteries age. Their structure is something like that of a garden hose. There is an outer coat which is mainly protective. Then there is a middle layer formed of muscular tissue. The inner layer, very smooth, offers no restriction to the blood as it flows through. Any obstruction in the blood flow would have serious consequences.

HARDENING OF THE ARTERIES

As we grow older all of us suffer to some extent from a hardening, or narrowing, of the arteries. It can become a kind of 'furring up'. A useful analogy is afforded by our electric tea-maker at home. It was given to us several years ago. Most people know the principle of the thing. It wakes you with a loud buzzing and at the same time siphons boiling water from an electric kettle into a teapot. Your tea is waiting to be poured into the cup. Ours worked well until one day we noticed that steam was escaping from the kettle and very little water was getting into the teapot. The instrument was dismantled, and it was found that the narrow stainless-steel tube which carried the boiling water from kettle to teapot was furred up, so that hardly any water could get through. The tube was cleaned and things went back to normal.

Something similar can happen to our arteries. But the analogy is not perfect, because the stainless-steel tube in the tea-making outfit was furred up along its whole length. With humans the 'furring up' of the arteries seems to occur in patches. This means that the blood may speed up after it has passed a narrowed patch, and so the person concerned may have no symptoms. During the Korean War it was found that, of the young soldiers who had died in the fighting, more than twenty per cent had some hardening and narrowing of the arteries, but they had suffered no ill effects. So this may start at an early age in all of us. The effect may be noticed because the condition worsens, caused by becoming overweight, taking insufficient exercise, smoking, suffering the stresses of modern living. But this we shall look at later.

BLOOD FOR THE HEART MUSCLE
The process of hardening which we have been

talking about is called arteriosclerosis. Sometimes we meet the term atheriosclerosis, which is used for the restrictive process in general. So arteriosclerosis is part of the wear and tear of life. In some people it is worse than in others. As a result, in these people part of the heart muscle gets starved of its full blood supply. The situation may not matter until the heart muscle is asked to do more than normal, and then the heart 'cries out for blood'. This is the angina pain. It may be all that the person concerned suffers, though it can be bad enough. The heart is asking for more blood – blood so that the muscle can work properly, blood so that waste products can be cleared from the body – and is not getting it.

Someone has said that the worst possible thing which could happen to a person suffering from hardening, narrowing, 'furring' of the arteries would be for him to eat a large meal, go at once into the garden and start digging in the hot afternoon sun, and then have a furious row with his next-door neighbour over refuse he alleges has been thrown over the fence. If he did not suffer a coronary thrombosis, he would have a very severe angina attack at the least.

We have seen that the heart becomes very distressed when it cannot get sufficient blood for the work it is being called upon to do. But worse can happen: blood may get blocked in an artery. Much will then depend upon which artery is blocked and how large the obstruction is. A tiny artery may only serve a small area. A block in one of the arteries supplying the brain can produce a cerebral haemorrhage; in the kidneys it can produce a form of nephritis; in the legs various circulatory troubles; and if it occurs in the coronary artery a coronary thrombosis occurs.

MORE CASES OF HEART DISEASE

There is no doubt that heart ailments are on the increase. Figures released in October 1973 for the United Kingdom were disturbing. They revealed that deaths from heart disease accounted for one quarter of all deaths in the previous year. Cancer was the second most frequent cause of death. In West Germany the figures were much the same as for the United Kingdom. In the United States the statistical returns for 1972 showed 361.3 deaths per 100,000 of the population arising from heart ailments. This was over one-third of all deaths. It was the major cause of the death of people over sixty-five years of age, but its effects were not confined to the elderly, and it gave great concern to the health authorities that early deaths were increasing in number. The death rate from heart ailments in men between twenty-five and forty-four increased from forty-six to fifty-two per 100,000 in twenty years. In Japan there has been a steady rise in heart ailments and this appears to have gone hand-in-hand with a more westernised diet; twenty years ago, when the Japanese diet was largely restricted to rice, fish and vegetables, deaths linked to heart disease numbered 34,298 in a year. Twenty years later, with a richer diet, they numbered over 70,000.

So investigations have been undertaken in a number of countries into arteriosclerosis, the insidious process which lies at the centre of most heart problems.

The matter of diet has been under close

investigation. Many years ago Dr Hugh Sinclair delivered a lecture which was to become famous. It was entitled 'Food and Health' and was delivered at the University of London to mark World Health Day. Dr Sinclair drew attention to the relative deficiency of the Western diet, and the excessive consumption of fats of animal origin. He referred to the hazards of the modern flour milling methods, which involve the removal of the germ in the wheat. A grain of wheat lying in the hand seems an insignificant thing. It is composed of three main parts – layers of bran, endosperm and the germ. The endosperm consists mainly of starch and comprises about eighty-three per cent of the whole. The bran is the outer husk and comprises some thirteen per cent. The tiny germ (some three per cent of the whole) is the portion from which the new plant springs. Today the bran and usually the germ go to feed cattle. But the germ, although so small, contains more than fifty per cent of all the vitamins and is the richest source of vitamin E (which, as we shall see, is of great importance). It is the most valuable part of the whole grain, but is eliminated during milling because otherwise the flour would not keep.

DEFICIENCIES IN DIET

Investigation into deficiencies in diet, and other causes of arteriosclerosis, continue.

In the early 1970s Alexander Leaf of Harvard University, U.S.A., visited Vilcabamba in Ecuador, Abkhazia in Georgia, U.S.S.R., and Hunza in the Kashmir, three regions where life beyond the age of 100 years is commonplace. After a careful study of the conditions in which these people live, Leaf came to certain conclusions, which can be briefly summarized, as follows: (1) the diet of the people in these three areas was low in animal fats; (2) the diet was moderate at all times; (3) meat and dairy produce accounted for less than two per cent of the calories consumed; (4) the air was free from pollution; (5) people were free from many of the anxieties and pressures of Western life; (6) they expected to continue working to a great age.

To test the theory that one of the root causes of this modern killer – heart disease – is to be found in our diet, a number of studies have been undertaken recently. At the end of 1972 the *Lancet* carried a report from Finland about an experiment in which over 2000 middle-aged, long-term patients in hospital were given a diet, some a normal one and others a cholesterol-lowering (i.e. low fat) diet. Each group kept to its diet for six years. At the end of this period the two diets were reversed. The evidence was that the cholesterol-lowering diet reduced the risk of death from heart attack by fifty per cent or more.

CHOLESTEROL

What is this cholesterol? It is a complex fatty substance which is vital to the human body as it plays some part in almost every tissue – one expert describes it as being like the mortar which binds together the bricks of a house. The level of cholesterol varies with the amount of fat which has to be dealt with. Some forms of fat appear to be insoluble in blood plasma, and cannot be burnt up by the tissues to supply energy. To make the fat soluble, the liver partners it with the cholesterol. These substances break down into tiny yellow pearl-like drops in the blood stream.

After a meal rich in animal fats, when an excess of cholesterol will be present, some fats may be squeezed through the arterial lining and accumulate on the wall of the artery. The droplets may increase in size. A bulge may occur in the wall of the artery, due both to the droplet and the irritation caused by the excess cholesterol. The blood no longer flows smoothly – it may silt up the artery.

A ten-year study in New Jersey, reported during 1973, involved 200 men aged between thirty and fifty. Each had already suffered a heart attack. Half the men were placed on a low-fat diet, and the others ate what they pleased. Again the low-fat diet reduced the cholesterol, and therefore the chance of a second heart-attack. Survival amongst those on the diet was seventeen per cent better than amongst those not on the diet.

It is obvious from these and other studies that cholesterol levels and heart attack rates are lower in countries, or amongst individuals, where the diet contains little animal fat. I shall return to this in the chapter on the treatment of angina by diet.

INCREASED SUGAR CONSUMPTION
Studies of heart ailments also point the finger of suspicion at sugar. Two centuries ago our forefathers ate only as much sugar in one year as we eat in two weeks. Even in the past few years we have increased our consumption of sugar rapidly. This, with our modern urban and city life, has spoilt the figure and the health of many of us. Our daily ration of exercise is negligible, so

the consumption of energy is low, but at the same time we have all developed a sweet tooth and the average intake of calories has increased. As a result many of us are overweight, and thus an extra strain is put upon the heart. Nutritionists have pointed out that heart ailments, diabetes and cancer are increasing all over the world and that this increase goes hand in hand with the increased consumption of bread from which the germ has been extracted, and refined sugar.

Other studies have shown that cigarette smoking has a harmful effect – one showed that heavy smokers are twice as likely to have a heart attack as non-smokers.

To sum up I use the recent report of Professor Jeremiah Stamler, who is Chairman of the Department of Community Health and Preventive Medicine, and Professor of Cardiology at the Northwestern University Medical School in Chicago. He states in measured terms that the Western world is undergoing a 'heart attack epidemic', and the World Health Organization agrees with this judgement. Professor Stamler says that the causes are 'a rich diet contributing significantly to the current high prevalence rates of obesity; the mass consumption of cigarettes; sedentary living and an increasing use of non/human energy (the motor car and television etc); and the stresses, tensions and conflicts of modern society'.

CHAPTER THREE

THE TREATMENT OF ANGINA

The treatment which has proved a very real help
to me is described in the next chapters. It can be
divided into three parts, each of which is vitally
important: (1) understanding oneself and the
stresses which bring on the pain of angina, (2)
medication and (3) diet.

1. Understanding oneself and the stresses which bring on the pain of angina

The first step in the process of dealing with
angina is to ask 'When do I get my pain? What
brings it on?'

We have seen how everyone may have some
thickening of the arteries, particularly after
middle age. In many people this is not sufficient
to cause any 'spasm' in the heart muscle, or any
distress. In others, the condition is more severe. If
the patient is relaxed, or working or walking at
an easy pace, the heart may get sufficient blood.
But as effort is stepped up, more blood is
required by the heart, and if it cannot get it the
pain of angina comes on. The heart cries out for
more blood. Many kinds of strain can bring on
this pain. Running for a bus, hurrying upstairs,
carrying a heavy parcel, walking into a cold
wind, going from a hot room into a cold one,
lying basking in too strong a sun, losing one's
temper, 'biting one's nails' with worry or
impatience – these and many other situations can
bring on the angina pain. The heart needs extra

blood to cope with the new physical or emotional strain, and it cannot get through to the heart.

It is all very personal. No two people will have the pain under the same load. But the strange thing is that the 'trigger level' remains the same for each person. In other words, the same burden will bring on the pain each time. It is at the same point of tiredness, or duration of effort, or amount of nervous stress, that the pain occurs.

So every angina sufferer has to sit down and work out for himself what causes the pain and when. Become a research student into your own illness. You are not going to become a hypochondriac. No one wants you to be for ever feeling your pulse, and anyway anxiety of that sort might bring on angina pain. But quietly, calmly, note day by day what causes you pain and when. Were you walking upstairs too fast? Did that argument at the office bring the pain on? Find the causes and try to avoid them. Take the stairs more slowly, determine not to be annoyed by people, not to get impatient, not to lose your temper. To work out this kind of programme for yourself, I have found, is the first step to better health and less frequent attacks of pain. To this I would add the practice of rest and relaxation referred to in Chapter Four.

2. Medication
Happily, both the doctor and the naturopath have ways in which they can relieve the pain of angina, and also prevent further attacks. These medicines should only be taken under guidance from your consultant – don't 'borrow' old Fred's tablets because they have helped his angina. Take professional advice, and follow it carefully.

One of the most valuable helps is nitro-glycerin (or trinitrine). The name may conjure up visions of explosives, and these tablets do indeed have something of that effect. They 'explode', or open up, the arteries and dilate the blood vessels, so increasing the circulation of the blood to the heart. The tablets are dissolved slowly under the tongue, and act quickly, bringing relief in about ten minutes. They are often the only means of instant relief, and many patients need to take them indefinitely. But they cannot be regarded as a cure, only as a way out of an attack, and the patient should lie down and rest as soon as possible. A tablet can be taken before some activity which may throw a strain on the heart. Some patients feel the need to take a number of tablets in a day, but if too many tablets are taken too soon after each other the blood-pressure may fall and the sufferer will feel faint. This will pass if he lies down for a while. Some people may have headaches during the first few days of taking the tablets, but these do not last long. However, a severe headache which does last, dyspepsia or any other distressing symptom should be reported to one's consultant. Aspirin will not ease the true angina pain.

The help of a naturopath can be most effective. He will use all-embracing methods of healing – herbal medicine (and remember that many of the medicines that the modern doctor uses were first discovered by the old-time herbalist) and other aids. A useful introduction to naturopathy is to be found in *Naturopathic Practice* by J. Hewlett-Parsons (Thorsons).

I and many others have found the following methods of treatment helpful, but I stress that I came to them through a consultant. *If your angina is anything more than a very mild variety, do not try to treat yourself.*

Vitamin E therapy

Dr Wilfrid Shute and his brother Evan, who are the world's foremost authorities on the therapeutic use of vitamin E, have found it to be beneficial to the heart muscle, and also in reducing the danger of coronary clots in patients already showing hardened coronary vessels. The primary function of this important vitamin is to reduce the oxygen requirement when a diminished blood supply, or the lessened availability of oxygen, is the cause of trouble. It has the property of dissolving clots and helps to ease hardened and narrowed arteries.

The Shute brothers claim to have treated more than 30,000 patients with astonishing success. No fewer than fifty-two per cent of those incapacitated with angina were so relieved as to be considered cured, while forty-four per cent showed a marked easing of their condition. One patient who had angina so badly that merely talking brought on pain now fishes and plays golf. In every case the Shute Institute insists that patients observe dietetic rules such as no salt, small meals often rather than fewer big meals, and a general slimming diet.

The Shute Institute normally starts an angina patient on 800 international units of vitamin E a day, but every patient should ask his consultant about dosage. Some 200 or 300 international units a day may eventually help him best. Caution is always necessary with patients who have high blood-pressure.

In the United Kingdom the medical profession looks doubtfully at the use of vitamin E for cardio-vascular troubles, even though its own drugs are often very suspect – one doctor listing suitable drugs for heart ailments mentions on page after page the side-effects which may be serious. In Europe, Russia, Japan, and Australia the case for the use of vitamin E is considered to be very strong. At the Fourth World Conference on Vitamin E held in Japan in 1970, seventy international scientists met and papers were read, all of which advocated the use of the vitamin as being more effective than many of the drugs used by the medical profession.

Vitamin E is taken in an approved capsule, obtainable from health food stores, but additional amounts (in small quantities) can be obtained from eating wholemeal bread, apples and vegetables. More information can be obtained in *Dr Wilfrid Shute's Complete Updated Vitamin E Book* (Keats Inc.).[1]

Vitamin and mineral supplements

The heart patient must be as fit as possible, and for this purpose a vitamin and mineral supplement may be taken. If it is necessary to go on a weight-reducing diet (see page 41), then it may well be that some of the essential elements of nutrition will be absent from the diet, at least in correct quantities. As the years pass, too, the body's demand for an abundant supply of all the vitamins and minerals needed for health and vitality becomes more urgent. There are a number of vitamin and mineral supplements,

[1]Distributed in the United Kingdom by Thorsons Publishers Ltd.

some designed especially for the elderly, and one or two capsules should normally be taken each day. Most chemists and health food shops stock these.

There are several helpful books which tell of the nature of these vitamins and minerals, and their usefulness. One or more of these should be found in most local libraries.

One last point should be made about the various vitamin and mineral supplements – these are not substances to be taken for a short period only. They are an essential part of one's food, to be taken daily, every day without fail if one wishes to be healthy.

Tranquillizers

It has been noted that sufferers from angina tend to be the thrusting, anxious type of person, always 'on the go', always trying to beat the clock, prone to worry. It is therefore necessary for the patient to 'slow up', and here we enter into a controversial realm again. Many doctors give this type of angina patient tranquillizers. Nineteen million prescriptions for tranquillizers were written in 1974, the minor ones in widest use being Librium and Valium. In one town in the Midlands in the autumn of 1974, there were so many prescriptions for Valium that all the chemists ran out of it and were without supplies for several days. These tranquillizers are used to slow up patients and to relieve anxiety, and in the doses usually given they are less likely to cause sleepiness than barbiturates. Addiction is also less likely, but alcohol may increase their side effects – which can be drowsiness, or lethargy, or blurred vision.

The patient who does need some help with

'slowing up' may be able to obtain this by relaxation, as described in Chapter Four. But there are several herbal remedies, with no side-effects, which can be used, and a naturopathic practitioner should be consulted about these.

Lecithin

Your naturopathic practitioner may suggest you take lecithin in tablet or granule form. This is obtained from the soya bean and is an emulsifier. Fat particles can act as the nuclei around which blood clots form, and lecithin causes these large particles of fat to break down so that they are readily absorbed through the arterial walls and therefore are less likely to clog the arteries. It is included by some manufacturing chemists in the capsules of vitamin E which they sell, and is also found in eggs, liver, nuts, cereals and vegetable oils. But we need to absorb enough vitamin B complex and magnesium to enable us to use lecithin, and here is the value of a general vitamin and mineral supplement. Cholene, which is found in most supplements, is a basic constituent of lecithin.

Pollen

During the past few years an interest has developed in pollen, which is not a drug but a food. Pollen is a flour-like substance, the grains of which are so small that they cannot be seen by the naked eye. We all know that as plants flower, pollen is transferred from the anther of a stamen to the stigma of a pistil. So plants are pollinated, some by the elements and others by insects and in particular by bees. Bees perform a truly remarkable feat, not merely in the distribution of pollen but in its collection. They do not swallow it up into the carrying sac as they do with the nectar; it is worked into a mass and carried in a ball between the hind legs, and so taken back to the hive. There are as many different pollens as there are various species of plants and flowers.

Intense research has taken place into pollen in Sweden, Russia, America, Canada, France, and Switzerland. At the University of Arizona it was discovered that antibiotics are present in pollen, and that it is the richest source yet discovered of vitamins, minerals, proteins, amino-acids, hormones, enzymes, and fats. It is thought that there are other constituents not yet isolated.

Interest first began in 1946, when it was discovered that more than 200 people living in Azerbaijan were over a hundred years old and still working, and that all were beekeepers. When selling their honey they kept the scraps from the bottom of the hive for themselves, and these were almost pure pollen. It was later that the discoveries mentioned above were made – that pollen contains vital elements in trace proportions, which appear to have a revitalizing effect on the human body, with no side-effects. The usual dose is about three tablets of 150 milligrammes a day, and these should be taken on an empty stomach. The best system seems to be to take one tablet on rising when the stomach is empty, and the others later in the day, at least thirty minutes before eating or three hours afterwards.

Strangely enough, pollen was valued long ago. Hippocrates, Pliny and Virgil believed that it assisted good health and warded off the problems of old age, and during the earliest years of the

Olympic Games athletes were fed on honey and
pollen.

A world-wide market in pollen tablets is now
developing, and new discoveries about it are still
being made. Ten years ago a Swedish hospital
reported that pollen would bring about a cure in
a high percentage of cases of chronic prostate
trouble. A Swedish specialist, Dr Leander, then
treated one hundred chronic cases, and nearly
eighty per cent were cured. These findings have
been confirmed elsewhere. Since many older men
with angina also have prostate trouble (it has
been estimated that prostate enlargement occurs
in seventy-six per cent of males over fifty-five and
at least thirty per cent of these are severe cases),
this discovery is important to them. And for
angina patients, the latest researches indicate
that pollen also has an effect in reducing
cholesterol in the blood.

3. Diet
Diet for the angina patient includes two very
important factors – avoiding becoming
overweight, and keeping to a low-fat regime.

(a) Weight and the angina patient
It has been stated by some nutritional experts
that half the people over forty in this country are
overweight. Modern life has helped to create the
problem. The daily ration of exercise for many
people is quite small – a short walk to the station
or the bus, some trips round the office. The
housewife may well get more exercise doing the
chores at home. But on the whole the
consumption of energy is small, and becomes
smaller the older we get, yet the average intake of

calories has increased. Calories are the measure of energy supplied by any one food, and a ten-stone man leading a fairly active life requires about 3000 a day. The number of calories required varies with age, build, and the amount of work done – from the 3000 or so mentioned down to some 1500 for a lightweight sedentary worker. Too much white bread and too much sugar has put up the amount of calories most of us take each day.

Does being overweight matter? Life insurance companies have no doubt that the life of an overweight person is likely to be shortened. They state that a person thirty to forty per cent above average weight for his build and age is twice the normal risk. His feet become flat, his veins varicose, his joints arthritic, and he is prone to chest infections and to heart failure. The last point particularly concerns us. The person who is overweight is asking his heart to do more than it was designed to do.

Studies by the Du Pont organization (covering thousands of people employed by them) have shown a fifty per cent increase in heart attacks amongst overweight people. If a man is ten per cent overweight, his heart, night and day, has to do ten per cent more than it should. Angina may well disappear, and life be prolonged by ten years, if the over-fat patient loses two stone. It may take two or three months to bring the weight down, but the diet will not be too difficult after the initial period.

How do we know if we are overweight? In one way it is easy to tell – the mirror will show us, our clothes will be getting tighter, we may become more breathless. Perhaps it is the waistline that tells us most. However, there are charts which can help. The best of these will show the average correct weight for build and for age. They can be obtained from your consultant, or from most chemists or health food shops.

In order to slim we also need a calorie chart, so that we may calculate the calories consumed each day. A housewife may need to cut her intake to 1300 calories a day until her weight is back to normal. A man with a moderately active task in life may need to cut his to 1600–1800 for slimming purposes. It is true that it becomes rather a chore to count the calories each day, but once you have begun you will soon get a rough idea of the number you are taking. Again, calorie charts can be obtained from your consultant, most chemists and health food shops, but I would recommend obtaining one or other of the excellent books now available on slimming, because your diet needs to be controlled and balanced. Just as a car needs petrol, oil and water, so the body needs three basic foodstuffs. These are carbohydrates, which are sugars and starches (these correspond to the petrol); proteins, which are required for both growth and repair; and fats. The body also requires water. All these factors are explained in a good book on slimming.

For those who are in need of simplified help, and quickly, I have found the following chart most helpful:

FOODS WHICH MAY BE TAKEN FREELY

Lean meat. Game. Poultry, but not goose. Rabbit. Liver.
Fish, cooked, steamed, but not fried.

Eggs, but not fried. Cottage cheese.
Green vegetables. Salads prepared without oil.
Clear soup.

Fruit, fresh or stewed, but not tinned in syrup.
Tea or decaffeinated coffee (with milk – see daily allowance below).
Low-calorie fruit drinks.

FOODS WHICH SHOULD BE RESTRICTED

Bread (not more than three thin slices a day). One and a half slices of crispbread may be regarded as equal to one slice of bread.
Potatoes (one average-sized one, boiled or steamed, but not fried or mashed with butter and milk).
Fats, not more than half an ounce of butter or margarine a day.
Milk, up to half a pint a day (this includes milk in drinks).
Salt – no added salt or salted foods.

Yogurt is a valuable addition, but should be restricted to the natural variety, not the kind which has fruit juices and sugar added. Many claims have been made for yogurt, and there have been those who thought of it as the secret of perpetual youth! There is some truth, however, in the theory that it assists the beneficent bacteria which are to be found in the stomach.

FOODS TO BE AVOIDED

Biscuits and all other food prepared with or containing flour, such as cakes, scones, puddings, pies, etc.
Sugar, sweets, chocolates, ices, jams, jellies, marmalade, treacle.
Fats, oils, thick sauces, evaporated milk, peanut butter.

Alcohol should be taken in strict moderation. A pale ale contains 150 calories to the half-pint, and two ounces of sherry contain ninety. Drinking chocolate and similar milky drinks are not good for those anxious to slim.

Gayelord Hauser, a famous American nutritionist, sets out his ideas about food in *New Treasury of Secrets* (Faber). He lists ten foods which he says are only fit for the 'garbage can': white sugar, white flour, potato chips, hamburgers, sugared cereals, cola drinks and bottled beverages, all artificial sweeteners, all hard cooking fats, frozen ready-made dinners, and overcooked food.

There is no magic way to lose weight. You must make up your mind to eat less than your body can use up in daily work, and it will then consume some of its surplus fat. But you must try to eat a balanced meal, and you should not skip meals. In fact, the opposite is now said to be true. There are many experts who can produce evidence that eating small amounts more often is better than having three bigger meals a day. Recent experiments with animals have shown that one or two meals a day lead to overweight, but five or six small meals not only prevent weight gain but enable weight to be lost. Large meals seem to tax the body's enzyme system so that food is not properly absorbed, and is converted into fat and stored. People who are in a position to do so might try five or six small meals each day. In any case, heart patients should never eat a heavy meal.

As the weight goes down the sufferer will find his breathing easier, and the pain less frequent when effort is expended.

(b) A low-fat diet for the angina patient

Apart from slimming, which will in itself ease the strain on the heart, is there any addition to or deletion from the diet which will help the angina patient? He or she may already be the correct weight for age and build, so what can he do to assist the heart by diet? The question turns upon the way the arteries are hardened and narrowed, and this we have already looked at. The role of fats in this process is of great importance. Fats can be of different kinds, hard or liquid: animal fats are mostly solid at normal room temperature; vegetable fats are normally liquid. Fats are changed by the digestion and pass into the blood stream, *often with excessive sugar consumption increasing the fatty substances in the blood*.

Excess fats may, as we have seen, be squeezed through the arterial lining and be deposited on the wall of the artery. It has been found that animal fats (called saturated fats) cause more harm than vegetable fats (called unsaturated fats). The latter leads to less hardening and narrowing of the arteries. At one time controversy raged over this, but opinion is now coming down firmly on the side of the vegetable or unsaturated fats being best in the diet. *The Encyclopaedia Britannica Year Book* for 1972, in its article on developments in medicine, stated that 'it is possible to modify factors believed to be involved in the predisposition to heart attacks. Reduction of one's intake of fatty foods, such as well marbled meats, and of cholesteral carriers such as egg-yolks helps. Cholesterol and heart attack rates are lower in countries where the diet contains little fat.'

Dr Hugh Sinclair, Reader in Nutrition at the University of Oxford, says 'Processing and

sophistication of foods have destroyed the
unstable helpful fats we need which are present
in such natural oils as unhydrogenated corn oil,
and have created stable harmful fats.'

The angina sufferer is therefore advised to
restrict his intake of saturated fats, and take
instead the unsaturated ones. This means
avoiding butter, cheese, fat meat, chocolate,
cream, ice cream, lard, and egg-yolks. But
unsaturated margarines may be taken, as well as
cottage cheese, egg-white, fish, fruit, skimmed
milk, and vegetables.

FATS AND CHOLESTEROL

Foods	Fat percentage	Cholesterol percentage
Meat, fish, poultry	38%	35%
Saturated fats	29%	6%
Dairy products	15%	16%
Eggs	4%	35%

Apart from the angina patient, *everyone* would
benefit from a diet lower in fats. Our high
standard of living, with plenty of fats and sugar,
is fattening us up for the slaughter. The
American Medical Association has said 'Fat
reduction in diet is probably of greatest potential
value to three groups: (1) the overweight; (2)
persons who have had heart attacks; (3) persons
whose own and family histories suggest they may
be particularly susceptible to hardening of the
arteries.'

What, then, might be an acceptable menu? I
have spoken earlier of a balanced diet, but what
sort of menu will give a balanced diet, keep
weight down, and be of a low-fat variety? I have
found the following most helpful:

Suggested menu (choices to be made from the following):

Breakfast

Half a grapefruit.

Poached egg, white only; or limit whole egg to one per week.

Average helping of grilled or poached fish.

One slice of bread, plain or toasted (or one and a half portions of crispbread). Unsaturated margarine upon it.

Tea, or decaffeinated coffee, no sugar.

Mid-morning

Tea, or low-calorie fruit drink.

Midday

Average helping of lean meat, poultry, liver, fish.

Two vegetables, average helping.

Large portion of fruit, raw or stewed, no sugar.

Mid-afternoon

Cup of tea.

Tea

Average portion of cottage cheese, lean meat, or fish.

Salad or cooked vegetables.

One slice of bread, unsaturated margarine upon it.

Large portion of fruit, raw or stewed, but no sugar.

Before bed

Tea, or low-calorie fruit drink.

One cream cracker.

At lunch a thin soup might be taken, and the portion of meat cut down a little if the patient is on a very careful slimming diet.

The need for roughage

Every diet should contain sufficient fibre, or roughage as it is also called. Today cancer of the colon and the rectum is a growing threat to Western nations. The reason is a lack of roughage in our diet through a heavy consumption of foods from which most of the fibres have been taken away. In Great Britain today the consumption of roughage is about a third of what it was a hundred years ago. This is not the place to go into a detailed examination of the reasons why a diet with inadequate roughage should lead to cancer of the colon and the rectum, and to a number of other diseases as well. But it is of interest to us that some experts are now stating that a lack of dietary fibre may be a factor in angina and in coronary thrombosis. In a survey of the history of heart ailments, Dr Hugh Trowell found a curious situation. Up to 1939, heart troubles had been increasing. Then wartime rationing led to the use of wheat flour with greater fibre content, and the trend was halted. The trend began again when the war ended and bread once more became the soggy white stuff we all know.

Laboratory tests have shown that when chickens, rabbits and rats are fed high-cholesterol diets to which fibre is added, their blood-cholesterol levels stay down. No one knows why. Other studies showed the same effect in humans. The addition to the diet of fats in high quantity increased cholesterol levels, but when fibre was added, the levels fell by twenty per cent.

These findings have been supported by the British Heart Foundation, who have stated that adding fibre or bran to the diet will definitely reduce serum cholesterol, both in animals and in mankind. The Royal Bristol Infirmary fed bran to fourteen patients between the ages of thirty-six and sixty-three, and there was a noticeable fall in the blood fats.

How does one add roughage to the diet? Wholemeal bread is a good source, and others are oatmeal, brown rice, vegetables, and fruit. But for many people who feel the need to add roughage to their diet, the best solution (apart from eating only wholemeal bread) is one of the cereals with the word 'bran' in the name. I find that two heaped tablespoonsful each day are sufficient. Cereal of this kind will also help constipation. It need not be taken with milk if one is anxious not to increase the consumption of milk; it is excellent with fruit juice. One ounce of such a cereal contains about eighty-eight calories.

Some random notes on diet
The patent slimming formula obtainable from the chemist, whether it is a biscuit or a drink, restricts the intake of calories and gives some bulk which fills the stomach and makes one feel full and satisfied. This may help to reduce weight for a while, but does not help for long because most people get thoroughly tired of it and return to ordinary food.

Weigh yourself on a certain day each week, on the same scales, and in the same clothes, or lack of them! Keep a record of your weight and you will be cheered by the steady reduction if you diet as suggested.

A walk after supper, even a short walk round the garden, is good for you. It is also good to rest for a while after your midday meal.

When out to a meal, do not risk eating or
drinking that which is forbidden in your diet.
Fortunately, slimming, even for men, is so
fashionable that your hostess will understand. It
may be difficult for those who eat in an office or
factory canteen, but there is usually a choice and
the right foods can be selected. A sandwich lunch
is not good for anyone as it means the
consumpton of too much bread: it is better to
take some fruit to the office.

Statisticians state that if the average person
takes only twenty calories a day above his needs,
he will increase his weight by two pounds a year.

People with what they call 'a sweet tooth' may
feel that if they cut out sugar from their tea and
coffee they must use an artificial sweetener.
There are two kinds. One is chemical –
saccharine and its variations – and you need only
a small amount to replace your usual helping of
sugar. These contain no calories, but I personally
would not use them. American and British
scientists have been concerned about all the
chemical sweeteners, and though the Americans
on the whole have cleared saccharine, British
scientists are still a little uncertain of the long-
term effects of taking it. The second variety of
sweetener is quite different, and includes glucose,
honey, and sorbitol. These give about the same
amount of calories as sugar of the same weight,
but are in fact slightly less sweet. Don't take
them and delude yourself that you are thus
avoiding fattening things.

Drinks
Since many angina patients are overweight, they

must be careful of their drinks. Alcohol must be counted within the total calorie consumption – too many people carefully count the calories in the food they eat but conveniently forget the glass of beer or sherry.

Regarding alcohol, it has not been proved, as some assert, that it will 'open up' the arteries and so ease an angina attack. It makes the veins in the skin dilate, it is true, and these carry more blood so that a person may get flushed. But this does not happen to the heart. On the other hand, anxious people may feel less troubled and more relaxed. A small drink on going to bed may be a useful sedative.

There is much argument about the use of coffee. A report in the U.S.A. describes the coffee-drinking habits of patients admitted with coronary troubles to various hospitals, and shows that heart victims appeared to drink more coffee than other patients. But it also shows that the investigators were not sure whether the coffee alone was the cause of the trouble, or that the coffee drinkers imbibed a great deal more sugar than the other patients. But if that was true, then those who drank a great deal of tea might be expected to be liable to heart attack, and this was not so. Finally, the investigators suggested that persons drinking more than five cups of coffee a day had about twice as great a chance of having angina or a coronary attack. So it is wise to limit your coffee drinking, or to drink a decaffeinated coffee. Health food shops stock a very fine selection of fruit juices which are very good for every patient. Mineral waters of the aerated kind are not good for those who wish to slim.

CHAPTER FOUR

REST AND RELAXATION

One consultant who specializes in heart ailments reiterated again and again to me, when I was at my worst, the one word 'rest'. Since angina is brought on by effort or by stress of one kind and another, one way to remedy the attack is to stop doing whatever it is that is putting a strain upon the heart, and to rest. If possible you should put your feet up; if not, then you should sit as quietly as possible, in a relaxed manner. Gradually the heart will be relieved of its need for extra blood and the pain will go.

F.N. Sutherland, a psychotherapist, says in his book *Teach Yourself to Relax* (English Universities Press): 'One of the most skilled osteopaths that I knew was a man who knew how to rest. With a very busy practice he certainly knew how to work hard, and I often wondered how he managed to do it all. One day by sheer chance I discovered his secret. I went to his consulting room, only to find the lights were turned out and the curtains drawn ... because a patient had cancelled an appointment, my osteopathic friend had used his spare time to rest stretched out on his own table.' If this was necessary for a busy man, how much more necessary it is for someone who not only has a busy life but a heart under stress.

So an essential need in dealing with angina is that the patient should heed any warning his heart gives, and at once rest. To try to carry on is like a man continuing to draw cheques when his

bank has informed him that he has overdrawn.
He ends up bankrupt.

RELAXATION PROCEDURE

The angina sufferer needs rest for the mind as
well as the body. It is no use lying down when the
pain comes on, and worrying about the pain or
the work you have been prevented from
continuing for the time being. To rest your body
whilst your mind is running round and round in
circles, pondering this and that, worrying over
things, fretting over inactivity while there is so
much to be done, will not really help the heart,
for mental stress is as bad for the heart as
physical. So we need to perfect for ourselves some
system which will help us relax mind and body.
Various ways have been suggested, and there are
books which deal with these systems in a full and
elaborate way. The following procedure is a
simplified one which I have found most helpful
and which may be adopted or adapted by
everyone.

1. Lie down on a bed or couch. Make yourself
    comfortable. Lift an arm, feel its weight.
    Now lower it until it rests on the bed.
    Concentrate on that arm, let it feel as if the
    weight does not belong to you at all but that
    the arm is sinking lower and lower into the
    bed. Do the same with the other arm. Rest
    for a few moments. Now raise each leg, feel
    its weight, lower it as you did the arm. Let
    the leg fall slowly, let it sink more and more
    deeply, as it were, into the bed. In time you
    will feel that there is no tension, no
    'tightness' left in legs and arms at all. They
    are sinking into the bed.

2.   Lie like that for a few minutes, breathing
     deeply and slowly. Now, whilst still
     breathing deeply and slowly, let each part of
     you go. Let your torso sink deep into the bed,
     let your neck and head do the same. There
     should be no tension in neck, back or
     shoulders. Let everything go. Everything
     seems to be sinking deeper and deeper into
     the bed or couch.

     Sometimes it helps to let the head roll
     slowly from side to side for a minute, and
     then begin to sink into its support. Imagine
     also that if you tried to lift up an arm or a leg,
     your head or your back, you would not be
     able to do so. It would be too heavy.

     You should now be completely relaxed,
     sinking ever more deeply into the bed. Make
     sure your hands are open, not clenched in
     any way. Ensure that no part is tensed.

3.   With eyes closed, just lie there. You may be
     inclined to fall asleep, but that will not
     matter. On the other hand, you may find
     your mind still dwelling on this and that
     which has to be done. Spend a minute or two
     thinking about something quite different.
     One idea is to think about some very lovely
     scene you saw on your holidays. Try to
     visualize every part of the vista. It may be a
     mountain scene in Switzerland, a loch in
     Scotland, a view of Snowdon, even a rose in
     your garden. Think quietly about it, enjoy it,
     and you will feel your mind relax.

4.   Now bring your mind back to today – you
     will soon have to get up and go about the
     chores. You are at rest now. Say to yourself
     several times words which will strengthen

and reassure you for the tasks which now have to be undertaken. Someone with religious instincts might repeat several times 'Thou wilt keep him in perfect peace whose mind is stayed on Thee'; or 'So long Thy power has blessed me, sure it still will lead me on'; or 'In quietness and confidence shall be your strength.'

The power of auto-suggestion has been emphasized by many people, and perhaps we all use it less than we might. We think thoughts of failure and despair, rather than thoughts of success and confidence. The non-religious person might well bear in mind the injunction of the famous Frenchman, Emil Coué, who suggested that we should say over and over again a phrase such as 'Every day in every way I get better and better.' This kind of thought, he said, should be repeated some twenty times. It will certainly, if it does nothing else, chase away disturbing worries and help us to be more relaxed.

IF YOU ARE AT WORK

It may not be easy to do the things mentioned above the first few times you try, but as you persevere it will become easier. And you will feel freer in both body and mind.

You may say, 'What about me, I have a busy life in the office, I cannot lie down on a bed or couch during the day?' Maybe not, though relaxation carried out as suggested before getting up in the morning, and when back in bed at night, is a great help. At night it will help sleep to come. But if you are a business-man, it should be possible to sit for a few moments in your chair,

perhaps after lunch, and make yourself
comfortable. Do not slouch, but let the body be
supported, and then let yourself go as suggested –
arms, legs, etc. Think of each part of you sinking
deeper into the support of the chair. When at
work, concentrate particularly upon the shoulder
and neck muscles. These get tight and tensed:
deliberately relax them. Think relaxing thoughts,
as suggested above. After a few weeks you will
find it possible to relax like this even in the office,
and just a few moments doing it will help you.
And, above all, do not forget the quiet, deep, slow
breathing. This is very helpful. Under the pain of
angina, try taking slow, deep breaths. When
about to face a difficult interview which may well
put you under stress, try a few slow, deep breaths
first. Under pain or stress, the breathing gets
quicker and shallower, so concentrate on this
aspect.

This system is only an abbreviation of many
methods of relaxation. If you are interested in the
subject you can read it up further. Some people
also find help in yoga, others in one of the
varieties of meditation. Whatever the method
used, the essential thing is relaxation in a restful
and peaceful atmosphere.

Tension is the enemy of health, and the deadly
enemy of all who suffer from angina. Relaxation
and deep breathing will not only take away the
tension, but also eliminate the fears and worries
which bring it on.

CHAPTER FIVE

MAKING THE MOST OF THINGS

It is to be hoped that the preceding pages have made it clear that, while 'angina pectoris' may be a grim title, to a great extent the management of it, the easing of pain and discomfort, the control of tension and stress, and therefore the amount of activity which can be undertaken, lies in the patient's own hands. *You can be really optimistic about the future.* You can continue to enjoy life. The last thing you must do is to think of yourself as an invalid. That will not help; in fact it will lessen your very real chance of living to a ripe old age. What you must do is to plan your life in such a way that the heart is spared as much as possible. To do this will not only prolong life, but it will avoid unnecessary pain and will help you to enjoy everything about you. So you have to wage a war, as it were. You have to discipline yourself to create such a regime, and to plan things around you in such a way that you can avoid angina attacks. I have already outlined some of the ways in which patients can help themselves, but in this chapter I deal with work and home life.

OCCUPATION

In almost all but the most severe cases of angina, the patient can continue at work. He may need a lighter job if his has been a fairly heavy task. If he has been a rent-collector or a postman, say, then he will no longer be able to climb the stairs or

walk long distances. The finding of the right kind
of job, if the patient has to change, may not be
easy but many employers will do their utmost to
help. Work of the right kind will be beneficial, for
idleness leads to brooding and worry and more
angina attacks.

On the other hand, the angina may have
developed later in life, near retirement. It may be
thought best to retire a little earlier than normal,
especially if pension arrangements are suitable.
But, again, idleness is to be deplored. Many find,
as I have done, that they can undertake a part-
time job with ease. Retirement, normal or
enforced by illness, is not to be synonymous with
idleness. It does not help any patient to sit all day
long brooding over his pains. And it will certainly
drive the other partner in the marriage 'round
the bend'.

So, many will find the opportunity to do a
part-time light job. Others will find an
opportunity to do some voluntary work, putting
back into the community without being paid for
it.

Hobbies are also important. This is the time to
take up new interests for which there has not
been the opportunity in the past. Hobbies
involving violent exertion are out of the question,
but bowls is a great joy to some. Swimming is
doubtful except where the water is really warm.
Fishing is one of the most relaxing of hobbies.

The thing which links all these matters – part-
time work, voluntary work, a hobby – is a sense
of purpose and usefulness. Busy people are
happy people. It is not just a question of killing
time; that which we do must have a purpose in it
and some satisfaction for us.

HOUSING

It may be necessary for a family to discuss housing. Some angina sufferers are unable to climb stairs easily, and unless there is a toilet downstairs this may prove very awkward. For some people it may be possible to move from a house to a bungalow. It may also be possible to obtain accommodation from the local council in a bungalow built for the aged or the sick.

If it is desired to move from a house to a bungalow, the question of removal to another area may come up. I found that great care needs to be taken in this matter. It is not wise to move, say, to the seaside where one has no friends. Shopping in a seaside resort during the summer may prove expensive, and traffic difficult to manage. One does not make friends so easily when older. If moving house, it is wise to take a good deal of time about the choice of locality, and the type of house or bungalow. Shops should be near and the roads should not be hilly.

THE HOME

Whether it is the husband or the wife who has angina, it is advisable to make conditions in the home as easy as possible. If it is the husband who has angina, and stairs are not a difficulty, either because there is a toilet downstairs or because they live in a bungalow, then the wife may feel that few changes are needed in the home. Fortunately, we live in an age when most of us have modern conveniences around us. But if it is the wife who has angina, it may be wise to make some changes. There are small things – for instance, a basket below the letter box in order to save having to bend to pick up letters and the

newspaper. If the patient feels giddy at times, it is
wise to have a handle built into the wall beside
the toilet, as this gives a good measure of support.
The Social Services Department of most local
authorities will advise upon such a handle and
other fittings, and some will install them free of
charge.

If the patient is very unsure of himself or
herself in a severe case of angina, a bath seat is
useful. This extends across the bath, so that the
patient can sit on it, and move his legs across and
into the bath. He can then lower himself into the
bath, or wash himself all over from the seat.

For the housewife with angina the distances
from working surface to sink, to cooker, to
cupboards need to be watched. She should be
able to do her work with as few steps as possible.
It may help to have the refrigerator raised on a
'dais' so that there is no stooping. A light and
long-handled dustpan and brush can be used for
the same reason. Cupboards should be low
enough to avoid stretching up far, as this gives a
good deal of pain to many angina patients. It is
wise, unless the angina is very mild and there are
never any feelings of giddiness, to avoid standing
on steps or a stool. To clean windows, a long-
handled mop is obtainable.

Polishing can be carried out with an electric
polisher, but it should be remembered that
slippery surfaces should be avoided. The main
problem in bed-making is the heaviness of
mattress and bedclothes. Fitted sheets are
available in nylon. Blankets can be obtained in
lightweight cellular material. Quilted nylon
eiderdowns are also light. Some patients find a
large sleeping bag easier to manage than

bedclothes.

Even if it is not possible to buy an automatic washing machine, a spin dryer is useful and much cheaper. It enables clothes to be dried almost completely and saves the need to hang them outside. After spin drying, they can be dried by putting them on an airer. For ironing, a board which folds flat against the kitchen wall is useful as there is nothing to lift. A fairly lightweight iron should be used.

I have already mentioned the Social Services Department, and this can help in many ways. The housewife who has angina, especially if she is a widow, might have meals on wheels, and there is much else which the officials of the department can do to make life easier and work lighter. A home-help can also be provided.

There are interesting leaflets available, varying from *Everyday aids for the disabled* to *Coping with problems in housing*, which can be obtained by those severely restricted with angina or any other ailment from the Central Council for the Disabled, 34 Eccleston Square, London S.W.1.

THE GARDEN
Unless one lives in a flat, the garden can be a great worry to the person with angina – except for those who do not care what the garden looks like of course, but then the neighbours may complain if it becomes full of weeds!

There are many things that can be done to make gardening easier. Expense need not be high if one has a son or a good friend who is prepared to undertake some of the work. If there is a lawn it is wise to buy one of the modern, very light, and quite cheap rotary electric mowers. There

are only two drawbacks to them – one is that
there is a long cord to the mains plug and the
gardener has to avoid running over this and
cutting it; the other is that the lawn needs
mowing often, and it has been suggested that
these mowers should be used twice a week. The
reason is that most of them do not have a grass-
box and therefore, if the grass is allowed to grow
long, when cut it collects into little heaps which
can either lie there looking unsightly and maybe
killing the grass beneath, or else have to be
brushed up which is going back to hard work.
Many people with small gardens will feel it best
to do away with the lawn, and have a patio in its
place. I found this a great labour-saving device.
Tubs of plants may be put on the patio.

Most gardeners, and not only handicapped
ones, are doing away with large areas filled with
bedding-out plants. Shrubs and heathers are very
labour saving. By shrubs I do not mean the old
Victorian kind which are associated with rectory
gardens and churchyards. A good nurseryman
will supply very attractive shrubs which, by the
use of different varieties, will give colour over
much of the year. Heathers are also able to give
colour in almost every month, and have the
additional advantage of forming, in time, a weed-
free mat. Some of them need a lime-free patch of
ground, and this can be given by digging out a
hole and filling it with peat before planting. But
erica carnea in all its varieties does not mind
ordinary soil, and will bloom right through the
winter and give a wonderful display in pink, red
and white.

Paths

There are a number of points which should be made about the garden and its paths. Not many of us would wish, even if it were possible, to redesign our gardens completely. The task would be too costly. But paths need attention. The reader with angina must be able to put his wheelbarrow to as much use as possible, and this will only be feasible if he has good paths. They should be wide enough for the barrow, and if made of bricks or paving stones these should be set in concrete if someone can be found to do this. This is the only way you can be sure they will remain level, and that weeds will not come through. Weeding a path is a chore that any gardener, let alone one with angina, will avoid at all costs. If a path across a lawn is required, then lay flat 'stepping stones'. They should be laid just a fraction below the level of the grass. This enables a mowing machine to work across them.

If there is a vegetable garden, a gravel or cinder path is possible, if cost prevents slabs being used. Again, paths should be as wide as possible to allow the free access of the barrow. If the garden is on a slope there may have to be steps, and these should be made wide and low with a hand-rail down one side. But where a barrow or a mower has to be used it will be necessary to avoid steps and make a very slow slope.

Avoiding digging and lifting

Of all the things which trouble an angina sufferer in the garden, apart from mowing, digging and lifting are the worst. Where possible, these should be reduced to a minimum. A lot of work can be done in a garden shed, working at table height, and there are many tools which will help.

A few general remarks may be useful:

1. Gardening is not harmful if undertaken with due regard to the effort involved in each particular task. Stop at once if pain comes on.

2. Weed control has been made much easier by the new discoveries of scientists. Weeds can be controlled for a year in paths, and in beds they can be watered with a chemical which will not kill the older and stronger things like rose stems.

3. Some gardeners have a theory that no digging is needed these days. The technique is to use a heavy mulch (two or three inches of it). The mulch of compost or of peat is put over the whole of the garden in the spring, and the earthworms draw this into the soil and so improve its texture. All weeds are choked. It is worth trying this method if you can afford the peat!

4. Clothing is important for the gardener with angina. During warm weather he will wear light clothing, but what is he to do in cold weather? If it is not too cold and there is a job which must be done, he should wear several layers of light clothing, not a very heavy coat which restricts his movement. But it is better that the angina patient should not work in his garden during cold weather, and particularly during a spell of cold winds. These conditions are very bad for him.

8. Planning applies to yourself as well as to the garden. Use forethought to limit your

walking. Have tools handy so that you do not have to keep walking back to the shed for them. A greenhouse is useful for the very keen gardener, because in cold weather he can still work there, and he will also be working without much bending.

So with careful planning a keen gardener, even with angina, can manage to provide himself with some gentle exercise. He will work slowly and rest often. He will certainly stop if he feels a pain coming on. And he will find enjoyment in the planned activity, and perhaps profit, too, if he grows some vegetables.

HOLIDAYS

Holidays are essential to most of us. A train journey is very convenient for the person with angina, so long as he or she does not have to carry a heavy bag. Many angina patients will find, as I have, that they can drive a car with perfect safety. They should, however, avoid long journeys and heavy traffic, as this builds up strain and tension. Allow plenty of time for a journey, so that there is no worry about arriving on time. Bank holiday motoring should be avoided! And the patient should make sure (by asking) that any medication taken does not affect driving.

A question which naturally follows is about air travel. In modern pressurized planes there should be no discomfort, but it might be as well to ask the advice of your naturopath before booking a flight. Ships tend to be difficult because of the many stairways.

Holidays, like so much else for the angina patient, are a matter of finding out what one can do without overtaxing oneself.

CHAPTER SIX

THE FAMILY AND THE PATIENT

On the whole, angina and coronary thrombosis are, or have been, mainly afflictions of men, though this pattern now seems to be changing. So it may well be that it is the wife of an angina patient who will be interested in these pages, along with all his family. What is said will, however, have a bearing on the wife if she is a patient. There is much the family can do to help the angina sufferer.

The ideal way to help is to create a restful, peaceful home. A happy and thoughtful wife is the best kind of doctor. When the husband comes home from work, he should not be greeted with an account of all the troubles of the day – the misdeeds of the children, the high cost of everything in the shops, an argument with the milkman over the accuracy of the bill. These cannot be avoided, but they need not be the first thing which greets the tired man as he steps through the door. Home should be a welcoming place. He will rejoice to hear of the successes of the day, the fortunate find in the shops, the good progress of the children. Let him hear of these first.

The man at the mercy of angina is likely to be the anxious and tense type, who does not find it easy to relax, and even on holiday takes some time to 'unwind'. He regards himself as indispensable at work, and probably he is. Or it may be that he feels he dare not ease up in case someone else gets his job. His restless mind does not leave him much peace. The wise wife will create a peaceful, relaxed atmosphere in the home. She will do her best to reassure and calm him. She will adopt an optimistic approach.

SIGNS OF STRESS

It is not so much overwork as stress which kills. To stress add a sedentary occupation, with a swelling waistline. And if to that is added heavy smoking and drinking, trouble is ahead. So a wife will watch for these things and try to steer her husband away from them. If these led to his first attack of angina, she will try to make sure he does not continue on the same lines. But she will lead him and not nag him. And when the better regime outlined in these pages makes him feel healthier and fitter, she will remember that he must not return to any part of the old pattern. If the angina was mild, then nature was giving a warning light and that must be obeyed.

It may not be too late to say – watch for predisposing causes of angina and other heart troubles in those you love, and guard against them.

The whole family can help – both in creating the right atmosphere, and in guarding against further trouble. If there are teenage children they may have to be told in a kindly way that records or the transistor on at full blast is not conducive to rest. Emotional strain has to be avoided as far as possible, consistent with fair play to everyone. This does not mean that one gives in to father at every point, but that one does not argue for the sake of arguing, and one learns to bide one's time and to make a point another day if he seems over-tired and under stress today. Weekends should be considered sacred, and not used to persuade the husband to rush down the M1 or the M6 to visit relatives or friends. They must be used to store up energy for the week ahead, and repair the damage of the week that is ending. This need not spoil everyone's weekend, however.

REST AND WARMTH

Whether the patient is still at work or has retired, it is helpful if, as far as possible, he can have a rest after his midday meal. The patient with severe trouble and not at work will find that an hour in bed is a great help. Winston Churchill was able to get through the vast amount of work he undertook during the Second World War because he went to bed for an hour after lunch. If it profited him, it will the rest of us.

The wise wife, or it may be the husband, will seek to ensure that the house is never cold. A warm house and a warm bedroom are essential. Angina pains can be brought on by walking from a warm room into a cold bedroom. Similarly, as I have said, the patient should not be encouraged to work in the garden on a cold day.

People with angina should not be allowed to get into a neurotic state, afraid to do a thing. If the husband is unable to work, or is retired, he should be encouraged to do a number of jobs round the house. There are many things he can do, and some he cannot. He may not be able to stretch up to clean windows, but he can do the washing up. He should not be sent to the shops and have to carry home a very heavy parcel of groceries, but he can do some shopping.

The housewife with angina can do much, too.

Some of the work she used to do standing, she can now do sitting. It will not hurt her husband to wash up even if he has shirked it in the past, but she can sit on a stool and dry things.

Idleness and mollycoddling are out. Life has to be ordered like a military campaign, so that what can be done is done, and all excessive effort which brings on pain is avoided. Limitations have to be learned and realized by all. But there is no excuse for avoiding all chores, all exercise, unless the patient is very ill indeed.

EXERCISE AND DIET

Exercise has been dealt with elsewhere, but this is always more interesting if others are involved. So let husband and wife take a stroll, even if it is only for a short way, after the evening meal. It helps to take the dog for a walk, but if he is the type which pulls badly, then let the fit partner hold the lead!

Diet has also been dealt with, but it can help the whole family. It need not be a case of father having one kind of meal and the rest another. Too many people are overweight, and every minute of the day the weight they carry round is putting a bigger strain on the heart than it should have to bear. And one of the serious matters disturbing schools today is the number of children who are overweight. So a wise diet can benefit the whole family, and need not be an uninteresting one. Try to get everyone to enjoy wholemeal bread, and to take less sugar.

Make sure the patient takes his various pills or capsules regularly. One of the biggest mistakes people make is to take their medication at first, and then to drop it when they begin to feel better.

Vitamin E capsules, and a vitamin and mineral supplement, were mentioned in an earlier chapter. Once again – if the husband is the sufferer, the wife will benefit from the supplement, and from one or two 100-international-unit capsules of vitamin E a day. Vitamin E is an excellent guard against degenerative diseases. It is also maintained by many that it helps women through the menopause, and prevents disorders in the reproductive system in both men and women. From the late fifties a vitamin and mineral supplement is excellent for everyone.

In heart ailments sex can be a problem, as sexual intercourse which is painful may bring on an angina pain. Great understanding is needed by both husband and wife. If one partner desires sexual relations and is not satisfied, married life becomes very difficult, and a further cause of stress is set up. On the other hand, sexual intercourse may be possible, and can be indulged in and enjoyed without pain.

The outlook for the heart patient has improved considerably. Patients can enjoy a reasonable, if not a vigorously active, life. It is noteworthy that insurance companies which a generation ago would have turned down insurance for anyone who had angina, or some other heart ailment, will now insure such people. Optimism is therefore the keynote for patient and family. This is the best medicine that the angina patient can have. Thousands of people who have angina are living very full and happy lives. This can be true of you, as it is of me. To live optimistically today is to make tomorrow easier, and life longer and more enjoyable.